MW00961584

# Gastroparesis:
# My Personal Journey

Patricia L. Rosati RN, MS, OCN

iUniverse, Inc.
New York   Bloomington

Gastroparesis:
My Personal Journey

Copyright © 2009 by Patricia L. Rosati RN, MS, OCN

All rights reserved. No part of this book may be used or reproduced by any means,
graphic, electronic, or mechanical, including photocopying, recording, taping or by any
information storage retrieval system without the written permission of the publisher except
in the case of brief quotations embodied in critical articles and reviews.

iUniverse books may be ordered through booksellers or by contacting:

iUniverse
1663 Liberty Drive
Bloomington, IN 47403
www.iuniverse.com
1-800-Authors (1-800-288-4677)

Because of the dynamic nature of the Internet, any Web addresses or links contained
in this book may have changed since publication and may no longer be valid. The views
expressed in this work are solely those of the author and do not necessarily reflect the views of
the publisher, and the publisher hereby disclaims any responsibility for them.

ISBN: 978-1-4401-1410-6 (pbk)
ISBN: 978-1-4401-1411-3 (ebk)

Printed in the United States of America
iUniverse rev. date: 12/19/08

# Author's Note:

I decided to write this book to detail my journey with gastroparesis from signs and symptoms to diagnosis to treatment modalities. It is not to be used as a replacement for your primary care physician, but rather as an educational and perhaps inspirational tool. This book will not be filled with graphs and statistics. It will be filled with personal information that I have experienced since my diagnosis in 2000.

I also decided to write this book to inform the public that such an illness does exist and how I was able to find treatment. Some of my experiences were good and some, not so good. My hope is that this book helps and offers hope to anyone suffering with gastroparesis as well as offering some insight for family and friends.

# Dedication:

*To my family with love. Thank you.*

# Acknowledgements:

There have been numerous physicians and surgeons who have assisted me throughout the treatment process. They will be mentioned in this book because I am grateful for their involvement and commitment to gastroparesis. A heartfelt thank you to Dr. John deCsepel, Dr. Robert Fisher, Dr. Sean Harbison, Dr. Daniel Cuscela, Dr. Anthony Auteri, Dr. Peter Andrews, Dr. Clark Gerhart and my primary care physician, Dr. Edward Carey. Thank you for dedicating yourself to helping others. Thank you for helping me.

# Chapter One: I have what?

Something was wrong one morning in September of the year 2000. I woke up feeling nauseated, bloated and wanting to vomit. Thinking it was just my nerves, I ignored the symptoms and began my day. After all, I was a nursing student in a bachelors program, on the verge of turning thirty, involved in a long distance relationship and working full time to support myself. It had to be my nerves!

So there I was, sitting in organic chemistry, when all of a sudden, I felt the urge to vomit come on so strong. I excused myself to the restroom and began vomiting. Knowing how strict nursing school is, I cleaned myself up and continued with my classes. Nursing school frowns on students taking a sick day. Ironic, isn't it. After my last class, I went to work. Still not feeling any relief, I called my primary care physician to try to get an appointment. Fortunately, there was an opening the next day. I couldn't wait to discuss what was going on with my body. After reviewing my signs and symptoms, my doctor referred me to a gastroenterologist. This is a specialist who focuses on digestive and any type of stomach disorder. There was someone in particular that my physician liked and trusted as a "belly doc". He even called him to set up the appointment for me. I only had to hang in there for two weeks.

I had two weeks to try to figure out what I had been eating that would cause such distress. I knew the doctor was going to ask about my eating habits so I thought I had better start doing my homework and do a diet recall. A diet recall is when you write down everything you have eaten for a specified amount of time. Between school and work, I really didn't eat a lot. But what I did eat was not that bad in the grand scheme of things. I ate cereal and frozen waffles for breakfast on most days. Lunch was usually at school and mostly tuna fish sandwiches or a slice of pizza. Supper, most of the time was a Slim Fast shake. I hardly snacked at night time because I was either too tired from the day or studying. My husband, boyfriend at the time, Tony, would make comments often of how I only have frozen waffles and Slim Fast in the fridge. When we had our dates on the weekends, he made sure it was out to eat or having a meal at his mothers' house.

Not really coming up with any great solution through the diet recall, I did scale back a bit. I ate more toast and cereal and less waffles, tuna and pizza. Now, I love pizza and I could eat it every day of the week. But, for this short period of time, I gave it up so that I could see if I felt better without it. I found out that nothing changed. I felt the same. Even with the extremely bland diet, I felt the same lousy way as if I were eating normally.

While waiting for the specialist appointment, I began to vomit more frequently and it did not matter if I ate or not. I was feeling bloated and nauseated almost all of the time. The day before the appointment, I vomited up some sort of blood clot the size of a half-dollar coin. This was my first clue that it was not just my nerves.

Appointment day with the GI doctor. Finally. I know I only had to wait two weeks, but when you are actively ill everyday, time stands still. My mother, who has been a ROCK through this entire journey, went with me. Tony worked in Maryland during the week and came home to Pennsylvania on the weekends. He obviously could not go with me. I will not name the doctor, due to reasons you will see later in this book, but he WAS labeled as one of the best in the area for any kind of "belly" trouble.

We began the visit like so many more to come by describing the signs and symptoms, intensity, frequency, duration and what makes it better or worse. Just like I suspected, he asked about my food intake. I explained my experiment using the diet recall and the types of foods I had been eating. He took my height, weight and vital signs. Then the physical portion began. As he palpated my abdomen, all I could think was PLEASE DON'T VOMIT ON THE DOCTOR. After a few more pokes and prods, the hands-on exam was over. At this point, he escorted me into his office to discuss my case. He explained to me that he needed to visualize what was going on inside my stomach. I was to have an EGD (esophagogastroduodenoscopy) to observe the tissue and function of my GI tract. I have never had such a test before, so I was scared. I was told that I had to swallow a tube with a camera on the end so my stomach could be evaluated. I was also told that they would take a biopsy as well. Now, anytime you hear biopsy, you think cancer. But, he explained that it is done to rule out numerous other disorders and not just cancer. Now, I know that I am a nursing student at this time, but when it is happening to you, you go numb. All I could think of was the fact that I gag on trying to swallow a Tylenol and they wanted me to swallow a garden hose. Then, some good news. I was going to be sedated! It is called conscious sedation. You are not really conscious but you are not under heavy duty general anesthesia either. It is a type of sleep where you are still able to follow commands but don't remember the procedure. The combination of medications received result in an amnesia type effect. That is one reason why you need someone with you when you have this type of sedation. They will be able to tell you what the doctor said because you will forget and ask over and over and over. The other reason for an escort is because you are woozy, tired and forgetful for the rest of the day. In fact, there is to be no driving or signing important papers for at least 24 hours post procedure due to the effects of the medications. That Versed is some powerful stuff! This was to be the first of numerous EGD's for me. Once the first one was complete, the fear was gone and I knew what to expect. On the bright side, I got some much needed rest anytime I "went under".

So, I made it through the test and it really was a piece of cake. I don't remember a thing and I found myself asking the same questions over and over and over. I am sure that I drove my mother crazy with that. The report showed a duodenal ulcer with decreased peristalsis (motility) in the stomach. Because of that finding, my GI doc decided that I should have a gastric emptying study to check the motility of my stomach and see if there truly was a delay.

Alright, so what is this test like? I was told that I would eat some eggs and lay under an x-ray type machine for approximately 4 hours so the emptying time could be evaluated. I could handle that. No poking or prodding.

On the day of the gastric emptying study, I reported to nuclear medicine and ate a meal of eggs, a piece of white bread and a whopping 4 ounces of water to wash it down. I was told that the eggs held a contrast in them for visualization of the stomach. Then, I proceeded to the x-ray table and was ready to begin a very L-O-N-G test. When the test was over and I sat up, I threw up. All over the place. Lovely image, right. But, if it ever happened to you, you know what I mean. After 4 hours, almost nothing moved from my stomach. The result, delayed gastric emptying. Better known as gastroparesis. From my research, I had learned that gastroparesis meant paralysis of the stomach. It is also described as a weakened stomach due to damage of the vagus nerve. Next step was to find the cause. This is an illness primarily found in diabetics. I was tested with the glucose tolerance tests and the fasting glucose and my sugars remained within normal limits. Another possible cause is scleroderma. I was tested for this and the result was negative. In light of all of that, I was now labeled with idiopathic gastroparesis. Idiopathic is the wonderful phrase used in the medical community when there is no distinct rationale as to why something is happening or how something has happened. Basically, idiopathic means, "we don't know". That's a comforting thought.

Having this illness, my GI doctor explained a special diet that I needed to follow to hopefully decrease vomiting episodes. It is simply called the "Gastroparesis Diet". It can be found through any search engine you try. It consists of bland, boring basic foods. Cheerios, plain crackers, Gatorade, broth, jello, low fat yogurt and water. Yummy. Well, there are enormous restrictions to this diet as well. No fruit or veggies because of the inability to digest them properly. Fiber is not a friend to people with gastroparesis because of the side effects. Believe me, I love apples, oranges, grapes and lettuce. I have tried to eat them slowly and sparingly, but great pain, nausea and eventually vomiting have occurred. I now am living on Cheerios, animal crackers and yogurt. Yes, I have lost weight. I will not say how much because there are some sick people out there that will say things like—"how do I get that illness" or "lucky you" or some other sick and twisted comment. Please be aware that not all people with gastroparesis lose weight. There are a lot of people who gain weight as well. It is not truly understood as to why, but it does happen and it is disheartening. Some theories revolve around the fact that for diabetics, there blood sugars become so erratic that the fat is stored. For others, possibly the malabsorption.

It is an illness, through my experience, that lacks compassion from many health care providers from doctors down to the bedside nurses who snicker and call you "crazy" as they are leaving the room. Having this illness, I believe, has made me a better nurse. I understand the physical and the emotional toll it takes on the person going through it. Take away a healthy persons favorite foods for one or two days and watch them try to handle it. We do not have our favorite foods daily, or if we try to taste them, it results in pain, nausea, vomiting, fullness and bloating. Believe me, I have eaten my pizza and shrimp scampi only to suffer after the fact. Sometimes it is within minutes, sometimes it takes hours until I vomit. The pain is almost instant but if you take away one of the greatest joys in life, what have you got? We use food for everything. We celebrate birthdays, holidays, graduations, promotions, dates, weddings and even funerals with food. Almost everything we do in society revolves around food. That is just the reality. Those of us with gastroparesis have to face a harsher reality. We take food and the ability to eat and digest for granted because the act of digestion is an automatic function of the body. When you can not accomplish this automatically, it becomes a burden on your everyday life. You begin to wonder if your electrolytes are out of whack and if you are going to suffer a heart attack because your potassium is too low from the vomiting.

You begin to look in the mirror and notice your hair is getting thin because of your lack of protein and other nutrients you are missing. You look at your skin and notice the gray and pasty color it has taken on since you are not absorbing properly. You look down at a round belly wondering how you have malnutrition when you are within a normal weight range. And yes, you can be malnourished and have a normal weight. Malnutrition does not mean lack of food. It means lack of nutrient dense food, lack of proteins and other vitamins and minerals that the body is missing. You begin to wonder, where am I, is this a dream or who am I becoming because you just don't recognize your own reflection anymore. This can and does lead to major depression and anxiety issues. Which leads to another problem. If you are taking meds for such issues and not digesting properly, how are the meds going to help???? They have a harder time getting into the system to do their job. Especially if they are not in liquid form. Therefore, many of the psychological components often go untreated. This makes the illness even harder to manage.

I will be honest with you. At this point, I was not suffering from depression. I think that was because I was so busy with school, work and Tony that I really didn't have the time to slow down and think about it. Having my mind pre-occupied definitely helped me through the beginning stages. It is true what they say, distraction is key in dealing with a chronic illness and symptom management. There is an old adage that my father would mention from time to time to help me with this process. He would tell me that he was going to hit me in the head with a hammer and that I would forget all about the pain in my stomach because my head would hurt so much. Funny, yes. Although I know it was not something he would actually do, he was just trying to make me feel better. As many people close to me did. I really did appreciate their attempts. It showed me how much they cared.

# Chapter Two: Now what?

I have gastroparesis. It took a long time to learn how to explain it, let alone spell it. Trying to tell people my stomach was paralyzed was and still is difficult. Especially with idiopathic. NO KNOWN CAUSE. If the doctors can't explain it, how can I? Here is the best I can do. Gastroparesis is a disorder in which food moves slower than normal through the stomach. Thus taking longer to empty and digest the nutrients. The term delayed gastric emptying and gastroparesis are used interchangeably. It is thought that solid food moves slower through the stomach due to some damage to the vagus nerve. The vagus nerve is a nerve that serves the head, neck, chest and abdomen. With the delayed emptying comes along severe, chronic nausea, vomiting, bloating, fullness of the abdomen, pain and early satiety. That's the easiest way I can explain gastroparesis without getting into too much medical mumbo-jumbo.

So, if we don't know what caused it, how can we fix it? This is a question that stays in the forefront of my mind every time I try something new. Why do I keep trying things that are "experimental" and basically "guessing" might work? Well, because if you have ever had the symptoms mentioned above on a continuous basis, you would try almost anything to relieve them. With that being said, I was started on a pro-kinetic medication. This is a type of medication that promotes movement. Sounds simple enough. Reglan was the first of many. My GI doc also had samples of Zofran for the nausea and vomiting for me to try. I tried this combination for about three months with no effect. Tigan was the next pill on the list. Kept the Zofran. Four months later, no relief. I had three emergency room visits as this point for vomiting and dehydration. I was told all sorts of things. Use your imagination, it's all been said. From, "you have an eating disorder" to "it's all in your head". But my favorite is still, "I CAN'T HELP YOU". This is a phrase burned into my brain and it was said by a PHYSICIAN. An EMERGENCY ROOM PHYSICIAN. What else can I say in regards to that statement. It irritates me to no end even to this day.

I remember one ER visit where I went to the hospital where my GI doc practices and asked them to call him for me. Fortunately, he was in house doing rounds. He came down to the ER and ordered an NG (nasogastric) tube to help decompress my stomach and hopefully stop the vomiting. If you have ever had one of these, you know that they are extremely unpleasant. My eyes are watering just thinking about it. It was my first and LAST NG tube that will ever be used on me (so I thought). I had to be the worst patient ever as the nurse tried to insert this tube. As she was pushing it in, I was pulling it out. It took three nurses to hold me down to insert the stupid thing. It was just so uncomfortable and you are expected to swallow as the tube advances down your throat. No numbness medicine or anything. Just up the nose and down the throat. They also started an IV with the antibiotic Erythromycin. This medication is shown to increase motility of the stomach. Hours went by and I finished the IV fluids and was stable enough to be released. NOT admitted and treated for the dehydration, but released to go home. You would think that vomiting so much they would want to re-hydrate me with IV fluids for a couple of days, wrong. I stopped throwing up long enough to get my discharge papers and out the door they sent me. I am still not sure if they thought I was a nuisance patient because I was there three times in a matter of weeks. Well, I couldn't be concerned with what they thought because they were not living this life for me. As a matter of fact, I was still working and going to school full time. How? I don't know.

Upon discharge from the ER, I was told to try Pepcid or Prilosec for the duodenal ulcer. The ulcer was not even on my mind. It didn't seem like much of a problem. The vomiting more than 5 times a day, nausea, bloating and early satiety—that was becoming quite a problem. Another follow up visit and another medication change. Toradol and Zelnorm. Supposedly, Toradol was going to help the pain and the Zelnorm was to increase movement. My GI doc thought that if it increases movement in the intestines, maybe it would help in the stomach. It didn't. After a few more months, he recommended a drug that was not FDA approved or sold in the United States. Domperidone. (Sounds like the champagne, Dom Perignon) I think the champagne would have been a better choice. My GI doc knew of a pharmacy near my hometown that could get it from Canada and compound it for me. Being non-FDA approved, it was not covered by my or any insurance plan. I thought that I would try it anyway because my GI doc said that he had heard positive things about it.

I began taking Domperidone once a day and I actually felt a little better. I reported this to my doc and he said to increase it to before meals and at bed time. Now, I was taking it four times a day. I felt some improvement. Finally, I thought that my health was on the upswing. Unfortunately, the upswing came down pretty hard after about two months. Even though it did not work as well anymore, I stuck with it anyway because my life was about to get even busier and I did not have time to get more tests or new meds. I was graduating and getting married!

In May of 2003, I received my Bachelors' Degree and was preparing for my upcoming wedding in June! At this point, I have been living with gastroparesis for three years and getting worse. As I mentioned, I had graduated with my B.S. degree and was planning on starting a Masters' Degree program in August. I told myself that I was going to enjoy my wedding day and honeymoon regardless of how I was feeling. Guess what? It rained on June 21, 2003. I was told that rain on your wedding day means luck in your marriage. I have been married over five years now and I believe that we have been lucky in our marriage. With all we have gone through so far---we are still together and I think we are stronger and our bond is tighter.

Our wedding was an intimate affair. About 75 people from both sides of our families and friends were there to celebrate. The ceremony was very traditional. After the ceremony, it was time to party. The reception was a lot of fun. Everyone was dancing, eating, drinking and having a great time. I won't bore you with all of the details because it was probably just as similar as every other wedding that you may have gone to. There was no great big drama and I was not a "bridezilla". It was just a wonderful party!

The next day, we were off to Jamaica. The first real vacation of my life! It was a flight that lasted a little over three hours and I was fearful at first, but then got used to it. Ascending into the sky made my stomach jump, but I did NOT vomit once on the plane! As a matter of fact, I did NOT vomit the entire week we were in Jamaica. I started to think that maybe we should move there because I felt so good. I know that stress does not help any health condition but this was on the border of ridiculous. I was so relaxed. No work. No school. No phones. No vomit. At the end of the trip, I was wondering what was going to happen once we got home and back to life. You've heard of Murphy's Law? Sure enough, the next day, I got sick with the nausea, vomiting, pain, bloating and early satiety. I can't help but wonder if it was just a fluke or something else?

# Chapter Three:  Still a student

August of 2003 began and I was working on a Masters Degree in Nursing.  At this time, I started doing active research online for gastroparesis.  I'm not one for computers, but thank heavens for the internet!  All I did was type in gastroparesis on a search engine and numerous entries came up on the screen.  One of the first ones I clicked on explained the illness and some of the treatments.  I was reading nothing new here.  Then I noticed a strange entry.  "Gastric pacing for the treatment of gastroparesis".  My first thought was, a pacemaker for the stomach?  I thought they were just for the heart.  I clicked on this link to discover it was for a procedure done in New York at St. Vincent's Hospital, Manhattan.  Being in Pennsylvania, I thought two-three hours away for treatment?  It was worth a phone call.  I finished reading the web site to discover that the surgeon, Dr. John deCsepel, has done this procedure with positive results. There was a phone number listed so I thought I would call and see what happens. I was pleasantly surprised when I spoke to the receptionist, Helen. She was kind and patient with my questions. She also knew what questions to ask of me. She explained how the physician works and gave me great directions because I was coming from Northeast Pennsylvania. She told me that the first thing I needed to do was to get my records faxed to his office. After they received them, the doctor will review them and they will call me back. I contacted my GI doc and asked for all of my records to be faxed. I thought that I was surprised by the receptionist being so pleasant, the surgeon blew my mind! He called me himself to review my records and discuss what he could do for me and this illness. Once I agreed to come to New York, he scheduled the appointment himself. I have never encountered a surgeon who does his own scheduling. Our phone call lasted about half an hour. He listened to all of my complaints and validated how I was feeling. He was the Chief of Minimally Invasive Surgery. I can not compliment his bedside manner enough! He always showed me true empathy and professionalism at all times. After I hung up the phone, I felt relieved to be going to see a specialist in the gastroparesis field.

A few weeks later, I was off to New York. My husband was able to find a new job here in the area and was able to have the day off to go with me. What a trip! We got lost! We were by the Statue of Liberty when we needed to be closer to Greenwich Village. Panicked at this point, I called the office on my cell phone and explained to Helen where we were. She reassured me and explained how to get there from where we were. Needless to say, we were a little late but that was okay. When I finally met Helen, she was as pleasant in person as she was on the phone. I had to fill out the usual forms as a new patient. She showed my husband and me where to sit and offered us a drink of water and the restroom. This was comforting knowing we came from such a distance. Once the forms were filled out, we remained in the waiting area for the doctor. Moments went by and then the doctor appeared and introduced himself to us. We went into the exam room and began. He first reviewed my records with me for accuracy and then examined me. Again, he was very professional and had a great bedside manner. I don't know about you, but I like a doctor who knows what they are doing and can be compassionate at the same time. When you are scared and nervous, it is a great comfort. It was at this time that I chose to tell him that I was going to school for a Masters in Nursing. After the physical, he took us into his office to discuss his findings and treatment course. He showed us a sample of the "Gastric Pacer". It was a strange little device with these wires dangling from it. My husband does not like medical talk and gets queasy easily. He was trying very hard to get into the conversation. I was just glad that he was there. The doctor then recommended another emptying study to verify the diagnosis. The test was done in New York so that the doctor could get an immediate report of the findings. Results did verify that I had gastroparesis. With the information in hand, the doctor began the process of gaining approval from my insurance company for the procedure. I am so glad that he handled the paperwork for me. The insurance company needed medical proof that I required this device in order to survive. It was FDA approved as a Humanitarian Device (investigative with a small population being treated), but the doctor had to prove the necessity by giving copies of the diagnostic tests, lab work and physical exam findings in order to be covered.

Going through this process, I was having blood drawn what seemed like constantly. From vomiting, my electrolytes were getting way out of normal range. It started with my potassium going lower and lower. Normal is in the range of 3.5-5.5. Mine started at 3.4, then 3.2, then 3.0. Each vomiting episode kept depleting my potassium. Once my potassium dropped to 2.6, my surgeon in New York STRONGLY recommended a jejunostomy feeding tube. He said that this could be done in conjunction with another surgeon while he is placing the stimulator so that I had a source of nutrition. We also discussed pregnancy at this time. The stimulator had not been studied in regards to pregnancy. Experts were saying that a pregnancy possibly could not be carried to term with the stimulator on without possible complications. My husband and I thought that we would turn off the device when we would try to conceive and use the feeding tube for nutrition. More about that later.

Back to my labs. I remember a conversation with my surgeon in New York. He saw the result of my 2.6 potassium and said to me, "I do not want to receive a phone call to tell me you went into cardiac arrest." My eyes welled up with tears and I really thought that if I don't get the feeding tube, I will die. This is not being dramatic, it was a bold reality check. Briefly, potassium works in the body to help with the contractility of the heart. If it is out of normal range, it can cause dysrhythmias, heart attacks and even death. So I had to think, get a feeding tube so I can have a baby or get the feeding tube to live. Naturally, I chose the tube to live. As much as I want a baby, if I am not here, what's the point? My husband agreed. He was definitely more concerned with my life over creating one. So we began to discuss the option of adopting a child. At this point, I was still too ill to think about it right away. We figured that we could just start gathering information and see how it goes.

Back to the gastric electronic stimulator also known as the gastric pacer. I was still confused about the whole pacer concept. The main goal of the pacer is symptom control. It has been researched and proven to decrease nausea, vomiting and pain episodes. It is not a cure, but simply a tool used for management of the illness. The term neurostimulator has also been applied to this device because it is believed that it acts upon the chemoreceptor trigger zone (CTZ) which is located in the medulla part of the brain. The thought is that the pacer sends the signal to the CTZ through the nervous system to NOT activate the vomiting response. I am all on board if the vomiting would slow down and the nausea eased up.

I am grateful that I am in the medical field so I understood what the surgery itself entailed. Dr. deCsepel was going to create a pouch in my abdomen and attach the wires to my stomach. The wires, or leads, are two insulated wires that are placed near the pylorus and will be connected to the stimulator. Once the wires are in place and the pouch is securely holding the device, I will be stitched up. There is an external programmer that the doctor will use to adjust the settings of the stimulator for the best therapy for me. It can also be turned off and on without the need for additional surgery. I will go into more detail about the programmer when I get to the chapter on surgery.

Being in school, I was limited to my time off. I chose to have the surgery on Christmas break. The doctor wanted me to have the surgery as soon as possible. I made the choice based on school and my ability to finish on schedule. My family has this running joke with me that I always seem to have surgery when it is cold or snowy. I have had knee operations in the past and each time, it snowed! So, why break tradition!

# Chapter Four:
# December 18, 2003

Surgery was scheduled for December 18, 2003. I had the pre-admission testing done in my hometown for convenience. This is where they do blood work, urinalysis, chest x-rays and EKG's. Once the results were in, they were sent to New York so that the surgeon could review them before surgery. Explaining the procedure to my family was very difficult. I know they tried to understand, but it was such a new technology that I couldn't explain it well enough either. Everyone was just focused on me feeling better. So, with everything arranged, my husband, mother, father and I got prepared for the trip. I had to be at the hospital at 6:30am so that meant that we had to leave home at 3am. My father had rented a mini-van of sorts to fit us and our baggage comfortably. My father was the driver and my husband, Tony, sat in the front seat to help with directions. As my mother and I sat in the back seat, she was falling asleep off and on. Tony did too. My father and I managed to stay awake. I was too nervous and a little scared. I mean, new technology is great, but when it is going inside of your body and you don't know how your body will respond, of course it is scary.

We arrived in New York with time to spare. It was very cold and windy in downtown Manhattan. Grateful that it wasn't snowing, just cold. It really stinks that our first family trip to New York had to be for surgery and not for sight-seeing and shopping! As we entered the hospital, the staff guided us to the patient admission area. We waited here for what seemed like forever. Once we completed all of the admission paperwork, we were taken upstairs to the procedure area. This was a large waiting room where all surgical patients for the morning waited their turn along with their families. My mother and Tony slept for a little while in this area and my father and I were laughing at them snoring. After waiting for about an hour, we were told that the operating room that was being used for my surgery was still tied up and it would be a while longer. The longer we had to wait, the more nervous I was becoming. I tried not to let it show because I wanted my family to think that this was no big deal. In reality, this was a HUGE deal! I was about to get an EXPERIMENTAL PACE MAKER IN MY STOMACH!

Moments later, they call my name. I had to go alone at this point and my family could see me once I was settled in the holding area. This area was where I got changed into a hospital gown and had to take my contact lenses out. I was able to wear my glasses until I was to go into the operating room. I was put in a cubicle and a nurse visited with me first to go over paperwork and check my vital signs. Then the surgeon came to see me and reassured me about the procedure and answered any last minute questions. Next visit was from the anesthesiologist. He went through a long question list to verify my allergies and previous reactions and any concerns. Not a stranger to anesthesia, I told the doctor how I vomit basically as soon as I wake up. He told me that they would give me something to help with that problem. Understand, the more nervous I become, the more I talk. At this time, my family is allowed to visit with me until they take me to the operating room. I am talking up a storm and going on and on and on and on. Then, I hear my name and here they come to get me. The nurse, surgeon and even Helen came to wish me well. I thought that was good customer service. Yes, I am about to have surgery and I am worried about customer service!

I walk into the O.R. and the first thing I notice is how unbelievably cold it is! I know it is for the sake of the equipment, but I HOLY COW it was COLD! Once I was on the operating table and they got me strapped in, they put these wonderful warming blankets on me. They use this machine that looks like a big microwave to warm them up. I would love to have one of those at home because I am always cold. So, here I lay, IV has been inserted in my hand and is infusing with something. I could not tell you what because I do not have my glasses on and I can barely see my hand in front of my face. Now I am just talking, talking, talking. About nothing really. Just blabbering on and on. All I can see are blue blurs that resemble surgical people. I hope they were surgical people. Then I heard, "Yes, Dr. deCsepel." I knew that someone familiar was in the room. He approached me and asked where I normally have the waistband of my pants. He said that he would try to place the device the best he could in accordance to my clothes. That was a personal touch I didn't expect. He was looking out for me in the post surgical sense. He cared about my quality of life. He then marked my abdomen to where he was going to put the pouch. Then the anesthesiologist gave me some medicine and that's all I remember! Surgery was starting!

# Chapter Five: PACU

I can barely remember waking up in the post anesthesia care unit. I do remember my mouth being incredibly DRY. I do recall asking for a wet paper towel to wipe my tongue and mouth. This went on for a while. Some time lapsed. I'm not sure how long I was in the PACU before the call came in that my room was ready. Once getting to my room, I had to transfer onto the bed from the PACU bed. When they were helping me transfer, I vomited. I am glad that I was still drugged up so I did not feel how much the vomiting hurt. Once I was settled in bed, my family came in to see me. Not really sure what to expect, my family approached me cautiously. They told me how great Dr. deCsepel was when he came out after surgery to talk to them about how it all went. He told my family that the surgery went very well and the feeding tube was put in without complications.

As the anesthesia was wearing off, I began to feel around my abdomen for the bandages. I felt a huge dressing that covered my entire mid-section. Then I saw it. I saw the feeding tube sticking out of the left lower quadrant of my abdomen. I was 33 years old and had a jejunostomy feeding tube. I know that it was medically necessary and vital for me to have it, but I just couldn't actualize it. Somehow, it didn't seem real. That is, until my first encounter with a nurse who came in to "flush" my tube. This is where water or saline is instilled in the tube to ensure that there is nothing blocking the tube. In other words, she was checking for patency. Now, being in nursing school, I have learned that the tube should not be flushed with cold fluids due to cramping in the abdomen. It should be flushed with room temperature fluids. My father and husband left the room when the nurse was about to begin. My mother stayed at the bedside and held my hand. She can handle ANYTHING! As soon as the nurse put the syringe into the tube and pushed the plunger----I screamed! She used cold water! Are you kidding me?!? I started to cry because the cramping was so bad and the anesthesia was wearing off so my abdomen was hurting. She apologized. I didn't know if it was for using cold water or for the fact that I was crying. Keep in mind that I did not tell anyone other than the surgeon that I was in a Masters' program for nursing. I didn't want anyone treating me differently. You will see an example of this later on. Once the nurse finished her task, she left and I never saw her again. My father and husband came back and they all stayed for a while longer. They made hotel reservations nearby instead of driving home only to return the next day. Once they left, I tried to sleep. The want to sleep was present but the ability was not. Every hour, someone was in the room checking on me. There were surgical residents and nurses who kept coming in to check my vital signs and dressings. It was nice to know that I was being checked on so frequently. After all, I was in an unfamiliar place. A hospital in New York. I knew the hospitals in my hometown because of my clinical rotations in school as well as my numerous ER visits.

Shortly after one of the visits, I recalled that I had not gone to the bathroom since I was brought to my room. I realized that I had a foley catheter draining my urine. They must have put it in after I was asleep because I certainly would remember someone doing that! I was glad that it was there. I could not imagine that getting up to use the bathroom would have been so easy.

Morning came and I was beginning to feel the pain in my abdomen. Two surgical residents came in to remove the initial dressing. Dr. deCsepel soon followed. He brought this briefcase that housed the programmer for the pacer. When he took the programmer out of the case, it looked like an over-sized palm pilot with this retractable little square attached. He had me hold the square over the incision where the device was and he turned on his machine. This enabled the transmission of data from the pacer to the programmer so that the appropriate therapy could be set. For some reason, I was expecting to feel something when he did this, but I felt nothing. He examined the site and gave me the green light to go home provided I could keep down the clear liquids and urinate after the catheter has been removed. He then said that he would be back after I had breakfast to review my instructions regarding the feeding and post operative care. The surgical residents then came in and removed the catheter and capped my IV. I did not need the continuous fluids anymore because I was about to eat! Clear liquids. How exciting---- JELLO. You know what they say...

# Chapter Six:
# There's always room for Jello

My first day post-op. Jello, chicken broth, apple juice and tea for breakfast. I ate about half of it and decided not to push myself to finish. Then Dr. deCsepel reappeared and we talked about the pacer some more. We discussed the different settings and volts and technical stuff for a while. To tell you the truth, I did not understand it at the time. I had to read the "Owners' Manual" for the device when I got home. It really came with an owners' manual!

After that was done, we discussed my feeding schedule and how to use the pump. He told me that I would get an electrical pump instead of gravity due to the fact that I was going to have to use it for 12 hours a day. Given my profession, I understood the pump. It is just difficult when you are the one attached to it! Because of my lifestyle, I was to feed myself from 7pm-7am. This was so that I could maintain as much of my quality of life as possible. The doctor also told me to increase my diet as tolerated. This meant to go from clear to full liquids and then to soft and then to regular foods. As I mentioned earlier, I ate about half of my meal tray and that was just enough to get me out of the hospital.

Then it hit me. I had to pee. I was in a semi-private room and I had the bed by the window. If you have ever had surgery before, you know that the walk to other side of the room to the bathroom is very long and seems like you will never get there. Sitting up was my first obstacle. It felt like it took forever. The nurse walked by and saw that I was trying to get out of bed and offered her assistance. I refused. I knew that if I was going to endure a three hour ride home, I had better try to do this on my own. That way I would know how I have to maneuver myself. I put the back of the bed up as high as it would go and swung my legs over the side. Breathe in and blow out and scream a little. WOW. I was sitting. Boy, the things we take for granted.

When I stood up, I could not stand straight. I was slightly hunched over. It hurt like crazy to try to straighten myself up. Deep breaths. I walked like this all the way over to the bathroom. After using the bathroom, I had to walk all the way back to my bed. All the way across the room! At the time, it was far. Once getting back, I literally climbed back into bed using my knees to crawl in first. It was the easiest and least painful way I could think of at the time. Guess how long this took me? Almost 40 minutes! 40 minutes to walk to the bathroom, pee and walk back. I adjusted myself in bed and felt a coughing spell coming on. I know that coughing and deep breathing help to rid the lungs of residual anesthesia, but what pain! I felt like my stitches and my feeding tube would POP.

Finally, my family arrived. They looked so refreshed. Remember that no one really got a good night sleep before the surgery. I was ready to get dressed and go home. Knowing that regular clothes were not going to fit, I brought my jammies. This leads me to a daddy's little girl story. Yes, even though I am in my thirties! Every year, my father and I go Christmas shopping together for my mother. He always bought me a little something as well. This year, he suggested pajamas for the surgery. The one store we were in had Snoopy fleece. Snoopy is my all time favorite and we were sold. O.K. back to the hospital. I put my Snoopy jammies on and was ready for my discharge papers. One of the nurses came in to discuss my restrictions on activity and diet. All of this I already knew because Dr. deCsepel and I discussed everything thoroughly earlier. I signed on the dotted line and waited for the wheelchair escort. The nurse also told me that the phone calls were made to have all of the feeding supplies delivered to my house. Moments later, the wheelchair escort appeared. Getting into the wheelchair was not that bad because I was upright the whole time. If you could have seen me get into the car. Well, that was funny and tragic at the same time. Once I was settled in, the rest of my family got in and put their seatbelts on. We were ready for the long journey home. Every bump in the road felt like my abdomen was going to explode. This was a very, very, very, long, long, long ride. My family kept apologizing for every bump that they hit. I knew it wasn't their fault.

On the way home, I had to pee. From having the urinary catheter and anesthesia, it is almost like learning to pee all over again. I had to anticipate that I needed to go so that we could plan our stop off of the interstate. The instant I felt an urge, I told my father so that he could find a place to exit. Getting out of the car was ok. Trying to walk into a place to get to the bathroom was hysterical. Again, I was walking hunched over in my Snoopy jammies and my hair was a mess! I can only imagine what the store employees were thinking when they saw me being escorted in to the bathroom by my family. I normally care about my personal image and what people think of me, but at that moment, I could not have cared less! I had to pee and I was in pain and I was tired and not to mention, far from home. After I used the bathroom, Tony asked me if I needed something to eat or drink and I asked him to get me water and I saw a single serving size of cereal and got that too. Cheerios. My diet staple. I knew that if I ate these slowly, I should be ok for the rest of the ride and hopefully not vomit. Just in case, I had my bath basin from the hospital right next to me. The little emesis basins that they give you to brush your teeth with are entirely too small to vomit in and I know that most of you would agree with me. As a nurse, I have never seen anyone capable of vomiting in such a neat and tiny little container. As a patient, I have never had the ability to vomit in such a neat and tiny little container.

# Chapter Seven:
# Merry Christmas

As I recovered, I was doing homework, lots of homework. Christmas Day dinner was held at my parents' house. Tradition. I wore my Snoopy jammies because I was still swollen and nothing would fit me. When you have abdominal surgery, they blow up the abdomen with air for better visualization. This takes a while to go down. My appetite was very slow to come back. I think that stemmed from the fact that I was so afraid to vomit that I would just eat very little and very bland foods. My diet, along with the tube feeding, consisted of animal crackers, jello, pudding and yogurt. The tube feedings were not going very well. In fact, they did not go well right from the start. Before I tell you about my Christmas feast, I need to digress into this story.

So, from the nurse who flushed it with cold water to being unable to tolerate the feedings, what an adjustment! The day after I came home from the hospital, my feeding tube supplies were delivered. Cases of feeding solution, bags for the solution, syringes to flush, distilled water, the pump and a pole. I was ready for my first feeding. It was to begin around seven in the evening. My mother was at my house helping Tony with housework and helping me get settled. I had the services of a home health nurse for as long as I needed one. I used her for one day and that was it. I was in the field and I felt competent enough to handle it myself. Yes—I am also quite stubborn. I let the nurse show me the first time and then I took over.

As I am sitting in my rocking chair with my first feed, I am waiting for the "sick" feeling. I had my trusty emesis basin, or should I say my bath basin, on my lap. I began the feeding at 60ml per hour as per doctors' orders. This made me feel full fast as well as nauseated, so I lowered it to 30ml per hour and felt better. I was not liking the feeding tube, so everyday I would try to eat more and more. I was still having a hard time comprehending that I really, truly had a tube to feed me, to live. I can not explain the merry-go-round going on in my head trying to realize the situation. Of course, I kept this merry-go-round to myself. I didn't want my family to think that I couldn't handle this. I mean, I have seen and worked with people with feeding tubes who were well into their eighties and terminally ill. Not thirty-somethings who still need to make their mark on life. Also on my mind was the fact that I felt as though I had to do as

much by myself as possible. I did not want to burden my
any more than I already had. To feel helpless is one of the worst
feelings. Having to rely on my family for my personal needs
really humbled me and put things into perspective.

Anyway, my intake was getting a little bit better. The tube
was giving me a hard time. As I was healing and the swelling
was going down in my abdomen, the tube site started to leak
slightly. Enough that I had to use drain sponges daily to soak
up the drainage and change them about three times a day.
Something else that I had to monitor. I had to check the color
and consistency. If it was thick, green and smelled foul, I would
have another problem. Infection.

Back to Christmas dinner. My mother's house is always warm
and toasty on days like this. She spends hours cooking and the
house is full of wonderful aromas. Not to mention that I love to
be warm! So we all gather around the table and as everyone is
starting to eat ham, potatoes, salad, cookies, pies and all of the
other Christmas goodies, I stare at my bowl of macaroni and
cheese. A toddler sized portion of mac n' cheese. Hey, I didn't
want to load up, I had a feeding coming at seven!!! Just a little
sarcasm. At least it was a step up from Cheerios. But, in the back
of my mind, I wanted a chocolate chip cookie. My mom makes
the best chocolate chip cookies ever!!!!!! And like you didn't see
this coming, I ate one. It was the best cookie I had ever eaten. I
didn't know if it would make me sick or not, but after all, it was
Christmas.

Christmas break was too short. Back to school I went. My class only had 12 students so everyone knew what was going on with me. We were a pretty close group. Everyone welcomed me back, including the faculty. The faculty at Wilkes University were very professional in regards to my condition, yet compassionate. My class was also interested in learning about the pacer and feeding tube. I showed a few of them my scars and the tube. I thought of it as a learning experience for everyone. I explained to them how it worked and I even let one of the students flush my tube.

Going to class was ok. I was sitting down. Clinical rotations were another story. Movement was hard still. It was only three weeks since the surgery. Moving patients around was not easy. However, I found a greater learning experience because my patients' knew that I truly understood how they felt. I would show some of them my abdomen. They would see the fresh scars and the feeding tube. It was actually quite beneficial for those who had or were going for a tube themselves. They saw that I was up and moving around and going about my day and that it was ok. I felt like I got a little more out of my clinical rotations because of this. Sounds crazy, but it's true.

I do remember one instance where I was doing my rotation at an area hospital and my feeding tube site started to bleed through my shirt. Just a small amount, mind you. Good thing I was in a hospital. I went up to my instructor and explained the situation. I was sent right down to the ER for evaluation. My labs were off, again. My white cells were elevated, red cells were decreased, hemoglobin was decreased, hematocrit was decreased. This was nothing new for me. They did an x-ray of my abdomen and it was within normal limits. They thought it might be bleeding from all of the movement and irritation. I was doing a lot of movement very soon after the surgery.

Once the ER gave me my walking papers, I went back to my rotation and finished out my day. I was beginning to act like this was all normal. Just another day in the life of a person with gastroparesis.

Well, school was going very well. I was healing and feeling better every day. I was also eating better. I was enjoying actual food. Minus the fruits and veggies. I still had to avoid them and I will have to avoid them probably for the rest of my life. Unless I want to puree them or make smoothies out of them. One could only take so much baby food. Because I was eating better and receiving nutrition from the feeding tube, my electrolytes were showing signs of improvement. Finally.

The one habit that I created was to cover my abdomen with my hands anytime I was close to something or someone. I was doing this for fear of bumping the pouch where the pacer was or having the feeding tube become dislodged. This is something I continue to do to this day even though I no longer have either one. It is a hard habit to break.

# Chapter Eight: Rule out what?

I had this wonderful routine of going for blood work after the surgery to see if my electrolytes were improving due to the tube feedings. Normally I don't recall getting labs drawn because it happened so often, but this time was different. My surgeon called me at home one afternoon to discuss my results. I knew they couldn't be normal if he was calling me himself. He started by asking me the basics of how I was feeling and blah, blah, blah and then he started talking about elevated white counts and left shifts and neutrophils and basophils are out of line and the eosinophils and platelets just weren't right. Then he said something that stopped time, stopped my heart and stopped the world. "We need to rule out leukemia." I don't really recall the rest of the conversation. To this day, I try to think about what was said and I can't. I just remember calling my husband at work, terrified and crying. His reaction was like mine. He was silent for a long time and kept on saying "what" and "you're not serious". He talked to his boss and came right home. His boss at the time knew many doctors in the area and was rather influential. He got me an appointment with a Hematologist/Oncologist within one week! (This type of specialist deals with blood disorders and cancers.)

When Tony came home, I don't recall how long we held each other and just cried in sheer disbelief. This can't possibly be happening now. I was just on the road to recovery. I think we were both in a complete fog for the week waiting for the appointment. We discussed it and I told Tony that I didn't want anyone to know about this unless it turns out to be positive. I could not possibly burden my family with something this heavy if it was negative. My family had just gone through this strange experimental surgical procedure with me and now I'm supposed to take them through this?! I could never do that.

Meeting the Hem/Onc was very scary. He was a kind man. A younger doctor who understood my fears. Tony and I just held hands as he went over my history and the notes he received from my surgeon and primary physician. He said that we needed to start with blood work. 14 VIALS OF BLOOD. Normally, blood work does not bother me, but after 14 vials, I was a little weak and light headed. They gave me a coke to drink and checked my vitals just to be on the safe side. Not only did they take all of my blood, we had to wait another week for the results. This meant another week in a daze uncertain of my future.

One very long week went by and I think that I had dried out my tear ducts. Tony and I went to the Hem/Onc and waited for the results. Very to the point, which is why I like this doctor, he tells us "negative" for leukemia. However, my white count is still elevated and the differential is still out of whack. The good news was that there was no leukemia to report, for now. He then recommends a bone marrow aspiration. This test was one of the most painful experiences. It ranks right up there with the NG tube! The object of this test is to get into the BONE and get a sample of the marrow. Now, the doctor numbed up the area really well, but you can't numb the bone. I remember Tony waiting for me in another room while I was on an exam table on my left side with a tear rolling down my face. I tried really hard not to cry like a blubbering idiot. This hurt. After the doctor was finished, he was apologetic. I knew that he was just doing the test the way that it needed to be done. I appreciated his empathy, but it hurt. Did I mention that it hurt? Tony and I left the office after a few minutes of the staff making sure I was alright. We had to wait another week for the results! We really were riding on the wave of optimism from the blood work coming back negative and hoping this would be as well.

Follow up from the bone marrow aspiration. Negative for leukemia. Whew. I felt relieved and very lucky. I could not imagine how I was going to tell my family that news. With all they have been through with me so far, I am beyond grateful that it was one less burden.

The doctor contacted my surgeon and primary physician with the results and they came to agree that my body is trying to get used to having a foreign body inside it. They explained to me the need to rule out the cancer due to the fact that the device might be masking something else and they needed to be certain. Of course, I understood. But, my mental capacities went out the window for a few weeks.

# Chapter Nine: Easter break

My appetite was improving about four months after the surgery. I was not vomiting much and my nausea was decreased. All in all, I was feeling pretty good. Surgery was a success. My surgeon was finally pleased with my electrolytes and other labs as well as my intake so he spoke to the GI doc who put the feeding tube in and asked him to remove it for me. This meant another trip to NYC. Not to the hospital, but to his office in China Town. My mother and Tony were ready for the trip. I don't think that I need to tell you how ready I was for this trip! It was decided that I would have this done on Easter break. Well, I decided this due to my school schedule.

We drove out to the hospital and parked our car and hailed a cab to China Town. It was amazing that an ambulatory surgery center was right in the middle of the fast paced area. We all go into the office, sign in and wait my turn. I did not have to wait long before they called me to come back to the procedure area. Again, the normal routine of vital signs, weight and medications. The nurse put the IV in my left hand and helped me get settled on the exam table. The GI doc came in and this is the first time I have actually seen him. Remember that I was already under anesthesia before he entered the operating room last time.

First attempt. He explained to me what he was going to do and gave me the wonderful drug Versed. As I was waking up, he told me that he could not get it out using the traditional EGD scope and he was going to try again with the colonoscope. The tube was in my jejunum which is why I think it wouldn't reach it.

Second attempt. More Versed and back to sleep I go. Colonoscope down the throat with success. Because it was my second time being put under, I think he went a little light on the medications. I woke up before it was over and I remember looking down my nose and seeing a garden hose sticking out of my mouth. I couldn't say anything because I also had a bite block in to help keep my mouth open. The nurse saw me open my eyes and react to being awake and the doctor immediately gave me something and back to sleep I went. The procedure was finally over and I woke up easily. While the nurse was monitoring my vitals, the doctor went out and told my family that the tube was out and I was doing well.

The doctor gave me the tube and I actually kept it in a plastic bag for a while to remind myself of what I went through and how lucky I am to be eating again. Being knocked out twice, I didn't remember much of the day. Though my mother and Tony told me that I was trying to stand up on the subway on our way back to the parking garage. For some reason, we didn't take a cab back and opted for the subway. I am glad that I don't remember doing that.

# Chapter Ten: Graduation

August 28, 2004 I was graduating with a Master of Science Degree in Nursing. Finally feeling pretty good for a change. I had made it through the summer eating slowly but surely. Maintaining my weight for the most part and exercising on the treadmill almost everyday. My medications remained pretty stable. The usual antiemetic cocktail.

Graduation day was such an accomplishment for me that there is no way to describe the pride I felt knowing all of the events that led me to this day. Before the ceremony, the nursing department held a brunch for the graduates and their families. I actually ate a little bit of the pasta salad and a couple bites of the cake. I was ready to cry over eating pasta salad.

During the brunch, the director of the nursing department handed out nursing lamps of learning along with our nursing pins with the year and our initials on the back. When I went up to get mine, I hesitated for a brief moment and all of the hardships, surgeries and obstacles that I had endured flashed before my eyes. It was actually like a flashback sequence that you would see in the movies! I could not stop smiling as I shook her hand and took my lamp and pin. I cherish these items to this day.

Once the presentation was over, we shared a toast with some champagne. Mind you, we were all adults of age and we were ready to celebrate!!!! Most of us brought a cooler with bottles of champagne in it and shared it amongst the group. It was a cause for celebration on many accounts.

Now that we were all feeling good, it was time for the commencement ceremony to begin in the gymnasium. We all filed in and listened to a few hours of speech after speech. Let me tell you, when you are graduating, you don't want to hear speeches. You just want your diploma. I remember sitting in my chair getting nervous about the walk across the stage. Why, I don't really know. Then the usher stood by our group and announced that it was our turn to walk. We stood up, proudly, and proceeded toward the stage.

As I waited for my name to be called, I looked out into the crowd for my family. Once I spotted them, I felt calm and ready to go. Then I heard, "Patricia Lee Rosati". I had some tears welling up but would not let them go, yet. I shook the hand of the University President and held on to my diploma for dear life. Once I returned to my seat, I opened it up to verify that it was really there. It was there. It was real. It was my name. I earned a Master of Science Degree in Nursing after all of that. My family was beaming. I could tell that they were proud of me. In fact, my parents threw me a party at their house that night.

Thinking back on it now, I do not know how I was able to go to school and do my clinical rotations while going through numerous tests, scopes, surgeries and feeding tubes. Not to mention the constant nausea and vomiting. The overall wanting to curl up into the fetal position and not leave the bed because of being too sick. Apparently, I wanted to be a nurse. I really wanted to be a nurse. I am a nurse.

# Chapter Eleven: Relapse

Time goes by and I pass the nursing boards and settle into work. I am still feeling pretty good throughout the next couple of months and eating small meals, but eating. Then, another change. It is now February 2005 and I am starting back with the nausea, vomiting and pain. A lot. I began to vomit daily again and had pain with everything that I ate. I went to my family doctor and asked him to admit me to the hospital with dehydration. He immediately agreed with me. I looked gray and sick. I knew this warranted more than just an ER visit. My doctors' office called the hospital and set up a direct admission for me. At the time, I worked for the hospital that I was going to be in so I got a private room. One of the perks of being on staff!

I drove home to pack a bag ready for a week of IV fluids and a clear liquid diet. I called my husband and told him what was going on and then I called my parents. My mother told me that she would come over to my house to give me a ride to the hospital and my husband said that he would meet us there.

Once I got settled in my room, my GI doc shows up to examine me and discuss what was going on. He ordered a HIDA scan. This test is done to evaluate the function of the gallbladder. It came back normal. Of course he ran the whole battery of x-rays and other scans to be thorough. All came back within normal limits. Three days of clear liquids goes by and I felt as though I could tolerate an advancement. Full liquids. I asked my mother to bring me a milkshake. Minutes after drinking some of it, I had intense pain to the point where I was going unconscious. My mother was on one side of me holding my hand and talking to me while my father was out in the hall looking for help. Like I mentioned earlier, I worked at this hospital! A nursing student was the only person who came in to try to help me! She got a cold wash cloth and stayed with me. I guess they thought that because I was a nurse, I could care for myself.

I could not believe that the nurse who was assigned to me did NOT come in to assess the situation. How irresponsible and unethical. Negligence. As a matter of fact, I did not see my assigned nurse for the entire evening shift of 3pm-11pm! And yes, the CEO and the rest of administration were made aware of this situation!

Back to my dad. He is out in the hall yelling for help and went up to the nurses' desk. They actually had the nerve to tell him that he was at the wrong desk for my room number. As a nurse, I KNOW and UNDERSTAND that any patient who is in need, I am to respond. After a little tension with the staff, my GI doc walked through the door. The next statement is the reason why I did not divulge his name. He said that because my HIDA scan was normal, the pain must be "MENTAL". He told me that it was all in my head! I don't think that pain so intense that I was pale, sweating and losing consciousness would be all in my head.

He then told me that he would repeat the HIDA scan but he didn't know what good that would do. I was totally infuriated that he would assume I was mental! He is a doctor. If I say I have pain, I have pain. You can THINK that I am mental if you want but how dare you tell me this to my face and devalue my feelings. Needless to say, that was the end of my GI doc.

The next morning, I had a repeat HIDA scan. I was also discharged after the test. I still think that my EX GI doc had something to do with getting me out of the hospital so quickly.

My primary physician called me at home that afternoon to tell me the results of the scan. My gallbladder was only functioning at 12%. It needed to be removed. I needed to find a surgeon in the area who would be willing to remove it knowing that I have the gastric stimulator in place. My primary recommended Dr. Peter Andrews. I saw him for a consultation the same week of my discharge and he agreed to do the surgery for me. He told me that he would try to do the operation using the laparoscope but might have to cut depending on the stimulator and how it looks when he gets in there.

Surgery day, AGAIN. I was told that I will be staying overnight because of my circumstances. The procedure was typical and uneventful. I woke up in the pediatric ward of the same hospital that recently treated me so poorly. This is because the surgeon operates there. I really enjoyed talking to Dr. Andrews regarding the procedure. He told me that he took some pictures of the stimulator while he was in my abdomen for his records. He gave me a copy. For me, they are cool looking pictures. For my family, not so much. Dr. Andrews has a great bedside manner and a very dry sense of humor.

I remember the morning after the surgery. I was getting myself dressed and ready to go home when he came in to examine me. He was surprised that I was doing so well and doing so much for myself. He told me that he had done a gallbladder removal on the guy down the hall and this patient was not even trying to get out of bed or do anything for himself. He asked me to go over to him tell him to get out of bed and get moving. This doctor has a great reputation with his patients and he was being funny, not mean. Please don't get the wrong idea. So, I walked down to his room and told him to get up and move. I told him that it gets better with every step. The nurse in me went on by explaining the importance of ambulating after surgery. I stopped myself and remembered that I had just had surgery too and I know how he was feeling. I wished him well and went on my way.

Along with my discharge paperwork, I was given a prescription for Compazine. This med helps with nausea. I had asked my doctor for this because of the gastroparesis, not because of the surgery. Keep in mind, that throughout all of this, I am still going to New York to have my stimulator checked. I am also still working and trying to maintain the best quality of life possible.

# Chapter Twelve: Not again

Late summer, I began to vomit again on a daily basis. Continuously nauseated. I have had the stimulator in place for over a year and should be feeling better, according to the research. I was not. I was feeling burning at the site and pain every time I bent over at the waist. This continued and in November of 2005, my surgeon started the insurance process to remove and reinsert a new pacer. He felt that maybe there was a defect with the device or perhaps my body was just rejecting it. My WBC's were still elevated. It took two months to get the approval from the insurance company to replace the stimulator.

I wonder if the insurance company understood what could have happened to me in the two month time frame it took them to approve the procedure. I have so many hang-ups when it comes to the approval of life-saving surgery and the insurance barrier. That could fill up another book. I am sure that as you read this, you probably have had some type of insurance issue yourself. They make me crazy. They try to dictate what a patient needs and what they don't. 99% of the folks I spoke with at my insurance company had NO idea what gastroparesis was, let alone the pacemaker. O.K., off the soapbox.

Another surgical trip to NYC. This time, Tony and I spent the night at a hotel about half an hour away from the hospital so that we didn't have to try to drive out at three in the morning. For some reason, I was pretty calm and not worried about the procedure at all. Even though there was a chance that the device was malfunctioning inside of me. I had complete faith in Dr. deCsepel.

Morning came quickly and we were off to the hospital. Same procedure. Go to the admission area and get checked in. Wait to be called and away to the holding area. This time, my parents showed up as I was in the holding area. Having been through this before, I did not see a need for them to go through another sleepless night again for the trip. Everyone wished me well and off I go, again. I don't know why people wish you well when you go in for surgery, the SURGEON is the one who needs the well-wishes.

Another cold operating room. I wished the surgeon well by telling him "good luck" and we both laughed. And then, lights out. Anesthesia.

I had a hard time in recovery. I just did not want to wake up. I think that my body was so worn out from procedures and anesthesia that I really needed a rest. As I slowly came to, I remember that wonderful dry mouth feeling again. This time, I had my overnight bag at the desk of the recovery unit. I had the nurse get out my toothbrush and I brushed my teeth with ice cold water for hours until the dryness went away. It must have looked crazy. Picture someone who just got out of surgery trying to brush their teeth with water repeatedly. There I was, trying to wake up, monitors on to check my vitals, can't keep my eyes open, can't keep my head up, in pain and I am trying to brush my teeth. It's pretty funny now. But, at the time, I was beside myself.

Surgery went well. No damage inside the abdomen. The device was intact but the surgeon had to send it to Medtronic for analysis. That is the company who developed the gastric pacer. They also do many other treatment devices like the cardiac pacemaker.

So begins yet another round of recovery. At that point in my life, I was a slave to the treadmill. I enjoyed walking on it daily. EVERYDAY. It gave me a strange sense of accomplishment to know that I can still get up and move around even though I felt like climbing into bed and not moving. Well, my husband and my father conspired against me and took the safety key. My treadmill won't work without the safety key inserted. They actually thought I would get on the thing when I got home from the hospital. Well, not the first day. Maybe the second. Just kidding.  If you've ever had abdominal surgery, you know that you could barely walk upright for a few days.  I may be a TYPE A personality, but I knew that I needed to recover and rest my abdominal muscles for a while.  I was a good girl and waited for clearance by my surgeon before I began to exercise again.

# Chapter Thirteen: Dr's without borders

At my follow up appointment, Dr. deCsepel tells me that he was going to work in Africa for an undetermined amount of time. It took me by surprise and I think I was in shock for a while because I don't remember answering him. Although I admire his decision, I felt a sense of loss because he was one of the FEW specialists who understood this disease and we needed him too. Sounds selfish, I know. We have been through a lot together and I was sad. I actually cried over this. I really trusted him. If you are reading this Dr. deCsepel, I am proud to have had you as a surgeon and I thank you for saving my life. Words are not enough to express my sincere gratitude for all you have done for me.

He recommended that I follow up with the Digestive Disease Center at Temple University Hospital in Philadelphia. I had no choice being the next closest doctor for this was in Kansas City!

I made a phone call to Temple and got an appointment with Dr. Robert Fisher who remains my GI doc. He is a specialist in the field of gastroparesis not just as a clinician, but as a researcher as well. Temple offers numerous clinical trials where Dr. Fisher has an active role. He is worth the travel time. It takes a little over two hours to get there and at first, I did not want to go. I was so comfortable with my New York doctor that I had this fear of getting to know a new doctor all over again. After some resistance, I have found Temple University Hospital to be a great part of my life.

The first couple of visits were rather routine. Review my history, symptoms and vital signs. Try this medication. Change that medication. I had a gastric emptying study done so that Temple had one on file for me. I also had a baseline EGD done as well.

Because gastroparesis patients are likely to have some level of reflux, Dr. Fisher wanted to perform the BRAVO chip procedure on me to measure the pH within the esophagus. This test involved implanting, lightly, a very small "chip" onto my esophagus. This was done using the EGD technique. With this, I wore a device that looked like a beeper that recorded pH at different levels and during different activities. Two days later, I was to give the beeper back so my results could be interpreted. While I was having this done, they also did an esophageal manometry. This test measured various pressures in the esophagus in regards to swallowing. I could not tolerate the test to be done the traditional way, which is via NG tube. Remember the horror I told you about in regards to that?!! So, they inserted the tube down my throat just before I woke up. This way, I was able to tolerate swallowing the tube without much irritation.

The actual test began as I was awake. I had to swallow as the nurse was pulling the tube out in intervals. I did not enjoy this at all!! I have a powerful gag reflex and I felt as though I was going to vomit every time the tube was advanced.

Alright, drama over. The test revealed that I had GERD. Better known as acid reflux. Now, I am on Nexium. In addition to Domperidone, Compazine, Tigan and Zofran.

I was told that the "chip" would release itself from the esophageal wall and pass through me system in a few days. I could handle that. But, one day, I was at work in the hospital and I thought that I was aspirating the thing. I had some chest heaviness and shortness of breath. I told my supervisor what was going on and down to the ER I go. They listened to my complaint and immediately did a chest x-ray to verify where the chip was. It showed the chip at the end of my esophagus.

I was told that the symptoms came about as the chip was releasing itself and trying to pass through my system. At least I knew it wasn't going into my lung! Back to work I went. Again, just another day in the life of gastroparesis!

# Chapter Fourteen:
# Botox where?

After numerous doctor visits and changes in meds, I was asked to try having Botox injections into my pylorus. What??? It is believed that Botox works by relaxing the smooth muscle. If the muscle is relaxed, perhaps the nausea, vomiting and pain would subside. Once it was explained that it would be done via EGD, I agreed. I knew that any treatment I was going to try would be experimental. There is no cure for gastroparesis at this time.

This procedure I have had done three times with no difference in symptoms. I am not certain if there will be any long term effects related to the injections, but I guess I will have to wait and see.

I am now working in Allentown for Sacred Heart Hospital in the Cancer Center as the Radiation Oncology Nurse. This position gave me a great outlet. I was the only nurse employed by the cancer center and one of my responsibilities was to continuously educate the client and their family as they came in for their treatments. Some of the clients were coming for months of treatment, so I really was able to create a therapeutic relationship with them.

It is through this position that I decided to study for and sit for the national certification exam in oncology nursing. I studied for months for this test. I enjoyed the work so much that I knew I had to specialize and become a certified expert. In the meantime, I am doing the diet of trial and error. I basically eat whatever I want and see how I react. Not a great idea, but I was hungry. I missed all of my favorite foods and wanted to go out to restaurants and EAT. I would do just that and boy would I pay for it in the long run! I would get so sick that I would vomit and have to go right to bed because it would literally wear me out.

Well the time comes for me take the certification exam and guess what, I passed. I am now considered an expert in the field of oncology nursing! I currently have the certification hanging up in my office along side my nursing degree. I can not tell you how proud I am of myself for that accomplishment. It was one of the most challenging things I have ever done. The best part is that my patients will be the ones to benefit from this because they will see that they are being cared for by someone whose sole clinical specialty is oncology.

The job is going great and I begin to have a wonderful professional relationship with the physician I am working with at the cancer center. It usually takes a few months for the doctor and nurse to develop the trust in each other necessary for patient management. Being it was going so well, I decided to let the doctor in on my gastroparesis life. Turns out, he understood more than I thought. He became a great support to me when I would be sick at work. He saw the signs sometimes before I had the chance to report them to him. This would lead me to a whole new concept of the "sick day".

# Chapter Fifteen:
# Working while on IV's

The period of time from April 2006 to August 2006 was rocky! I was very fortunate to work with a physician who understood my problem. Radiation Oncologist, Dr. Daniel Cuscela. He has a strong research background and he was always looking up information for me. Anytime I came to work and was vomiting, he sent me up to the Short Stay Procedure Unit for IV fluids. It got to a point where I was receiving lipids and IV fluids at least twice a week. This did help to get me through the days. Like I mentioned previously, a new meaning of the word, "sick day". He would also call the GI doc there and get me earlier appointments.

I tried the Botox again in August with Dr. Auteri at Sacred Heart Hospital. Being an EGD was being done, so was another biopsy. They do this to examine the tissue for any abnormalities. This time, they found a small hiatal hernia and something I was not expecting. Barrett's Esophagus. I asked for my medical record of this test. I like to see it for myself and keep it for my records. Working in the oncology field, I had access to the pathologists. I showed them the report and they explained that Barrett's is where the cells are abnormal; whether they are in a state of metaplasia or dysplasia.

Basically, it is considered a pre-cancerous condition where surveillance EGD's are done on a routine basis to watch for changes in the tissue. Should the cells become dysplasic, esophageal cancer may develop. My cells at that time were metaplasia cells and I would be getting annual EGD's for monitoring. This is something that I MUST monitor so that in the event they turn cancerous, I should catch it early enough for successful treatment.

In my mind, I am putting all of this together. I was tested for leukemia. Negative. I am an Oncology Certified Nurse. Ironic. Now, I may develop esophageal cancer. Fantastic. I sometimes wonder if the past lab results and leukemia scare were a precursor to this. The more you learn, you can't help but analyze every little detail. Sometimes that could be good, sometimes that could be bad. The focus should be on me living my best life possible, not focusing on the minute details that prevent me from doing so.

My medication cocktail now consists of Nexium, Domperidone, Zofran, Compazine, Tigan and the occasional Excedrin PM to help me sleep. My diet remains pretty sketchy. I want the same freedoms that my friends and family have when it comes to food so I take my chances sometimes and eat whatever I feel like. I deal with the postprandial problems just like it was a normal part of my life. I feel the wave of nausea, vomit and then get back to what I was doing. It has become a very strange routine that I am sure a lot of people with gastroparesis can attest to.

# Chapter Sixteen:
# Chronic infection

In November of 2006, I had a routine follow up visit with Dr. Fisher at Temple. Still having the nausea, vomiting, bloating and early satiety. My white blood cells also remained elevated. Still. It was reviewed between myself, Dr. Fisher and surgeon, Dr. Harbison and it was time for the stimulator to come out. Dr. Harbison was going to do the procedure along with performing a pyloroplasty at the same time.

A pyloroplasty is where the opening of the pylorus is surgically manipulated to widen the pyloric valve; thus helping with the emptying of the stomach contents. Well, I had no choice. O.K. Sign me up.

At this time, I was between jobs because of my illness. I was to start a new job in January of 2007 as a Clinical Nurse Specialist in Oncology.

December 8, 2006. Surgery day, again. What a broken record I have become. This was my first major procedure at Temple, but I wasn't nervous. It seems strange to say, but it was almost a routine part of my life.

The admissions procedure is basically the same anywhere you go. Lab tests, checking in, vital signs, IVs, hospital gowns and waiting for your turn. I was taken to the OR wide awake and not really nervous. Dr. Harbison explained once again what he was going to do and as anesthesia was about to begin their medication administration, I became nervous. I started to ramble on and on and on. Then, something totally surprising happened. Dr. Harbison actually held my hand as if to offer me assurance that everything would be alright. I remember a warm feeling of contentment and off to sleep I went.

Surgery went well and the device was out. Pyloroplasty complete. I woke up in a private room on the bariatric wing of the hospital. I thought that was odd but it may have been the only place available at the time. I really appreciated the private room. I know that a lot of hospitals are trying to become all private to help decrease the risk of infection, which we really need. I am not sure if that was the reason why I was alone. I did not ask.

That evening, I was up and out of bed walking in the halls and getting myself to the bathroom without much trouble. My family drove home that day and it was decided that only Tony would return to pick me up. This surgery was a piece of cake in comparison so I really didn't need the entourage.

I slept really well that night and woke up refreshed and ready to go home. I ate the usual clear liquid diet and did some laps around the nurses' station. Dr. Harbison was in early in the morning and wrote my discharge orders. I had four small stab wounds and one large incision on my abdomen. The incision was from where the pacer was. Because it was under my skin in a pouch, he needed to cut in order to reach it. So again I had to deal with the coughing spells and practice my deep breathing.

The pain was not that bad and I have a tendency to not take anything stronger than a Tylenol for pain. Narcotics slow down the motility of the stomach and cause constipation. Not a problem needed for someone who already has those issues. I think that I may have mentioned that once before. I repeat myself so often with this illness that I lose a piece of my mind every time. Those of you with problem can relate.

Tony shows up at the hospital and it is time to hit the road. The ride was not that bad. Once we got to the PA Turnpike, it went pretty smooth. The stop-and-go Philly traffic was a bit much to handle. We made it home safe and sound and I began to recover, again.

# Chapter Seventeen: Try again

Time went on and I still was not having relief from the nausea and vomiting. It was felt that maybe the pylorus was not open enough. Since then, there have been good days and bad days. I really try not to tell my family too much. Burden. Everything that I was eating at this time was hurting and giving me unrelenting nausea. I was vomiting at least twice a day and regurgitating often. I know that I have GERD and a hiatal hernia and Barretts's Esophagus along with the gastroparesis, but I just want to feel NORMAL! I want to feel like I could go out to eat with my husband and not feel like I am wasting money on food because I will vomit when we get home. Sometimes, I vomit before we even leave the restaurant. It is now March of 2007 and I am still working full time. I am nauseated ALL of the time. I don't want to eat because it hurts my abdominal area so much. Not only does food hurt, my abdomen distends almost immediately after swallowing any food.

I can't find a pattern of what food make it worse. Eggs, toast, cheerios—I tolerate well. Not a day goes by when I don't think of that J-tube coming back because my electrolytes are so off due to malabsorption.

Yet another appointment with my GI doc and he recommends something called a balloon dilatation. This is where they perform an EGD and utilize three different size balloons to expand the opening of the pylorus by gently inflating them and stretching out the muscle. All three balloons are used and after the procedure, they are deflated and removed, hopefully offering some sense of relief.

My next appointment was in May and my husband got the day off of work to travel to Philly with me. After the usual routine of weight and vital signs, the doc comes in and we begin to review my signs and symptoms. I told him how great I felt for almost two months post dilatation, but unfortunately, the symptoms are coming back in full force. He quickly told me that the dilatation procedure could be done again. I agreed. Then he mentioned to me a clinical trial that may be on the horizon soon. At this time, not much is known about it, but it is supposed to help with abdominal pain. I had asked to be put on the list for consideration whenever it becomes available.

June 13 was another balloon dilatation day! Here we go again. More sedation. Another EGD. I feel like I could do the test myself! The staff in the Endoscopy Suite really recognized me now. It feels really good to be greeted and comforted by them, but I would rather see them out at a restaurant instead of at the hospital. My husband escorted me to the procedure this time. Usually, it is my mother who goes with me. I am glad that Tony went so he could understand what was involved with this. He was actually quite calm for someone who is NOT in any way interested in the medical field. I admit that I was a bit nervous. Not over the EGD, but over the "what-ifs". I'm tired. I'm tired of telling everyone the same complaints over and over. I'm tired of explaining over and over. I'm tired of justifying my food intake. I'm tired of explaining where, when and how much I ate. I know that people are just asking out of concern, but it is exhausting! I just want to be normal to some extent. You don't realize how your stomach works until it doesn't. You don't realize how much you love food and dinner with friends and family until you can't enjoy it anymore. It is truly amazing what we take for granted. We wake up everyday and ASSUME our bodies will work and function normally.

Again, I have about two months of "better days" after the balloon dilatation. I am still on the bland and boring diet. I call to schedule a check-up with my GI doc. This time, I travel alone. I don't mind. It is just an office visit. This visit was different. I explained how I was not improving and how I was feeling worse. My doctor didn't have anymore options for me at this time except for the J-tube to come back into my life. I left after I told him that I really needed to think about it.

The drive home was a very long two hours. I kept thinking about the "tube". I actually refer to it as "that stupid tube". I know. Very mature. Remember, in the beginning of the book, I mentioned adoption. Well, my husband and I were getting closer to completing our International Adoption from China and would I really want to have a feeding tube while traveling or better yet, while trying to raise my child??

# Chapter Eighteen: The letter

One day in August, I received a letter. August 20, 2007 to be exact. It was from my GI doc at Temple. He explained that there are currently NO MORE options for me at this time regarding gastroparesis and symptom management. His only recommendation was for the jejunostomy feeding tube. It was like reliving the office visit all over again. This time, it was in black and white. It went on to say that I could just call him back and he would do a direct admit to the hospital or if I needed another office visit, we could do that also. Stunned. I never called him back regarding that letter.

After stewing for a bit over the letter, I continued to have appointments with my doc at Temple. Mostly because I knew that Dr. Fisher was the best and I really was in good hands. I just needed some time to absorb the reality of my situation. I was not eating well. I was vomiting. I was nauseated. I was dehydrated. I was in pain. I was bloated. I was tired.

I kept plugging away at work and at life. I could only sit around and feel sorry for myself for so long. Yes, there have been many times that I have cornered myself off from the world and just cried. But in front of people, the act would be on. My game-face would be on in full force.

At work, people would tell me that I looked gray or that I looked sick. Well, unfortunately I could not hide that. My hair was still falling out. In clumps. People at work noticed that too. I often wondered why people couldn't focus on me as a person, not the girl with gastroparesis.

I had so many people ask me why I was not trying to get some sort of Disability or Social Security. I knew that I would be eligible. My answer was simple. As long as I am able to get out of bed, I don't need it. Everyone has to modify their life in one way or another to accommodate some type of situation. Whether it be an illness, a loved one, a career or school. There are numerous examples. I had just learned to modify my life to a point where it became second nature. It really stinks to say it, but you learn how to deal and move on.

# Chapter Nineteen: Dehydration anyone

In September, I was feeling really yucky. Nauseated all of the time, vomiting—a lot!!! I was weak, tired, irritable and just plain sick. I called my primary care physician and requested a same day appointment.

The minute he saw me, he said that I needed to be admitted. Again, I was gray and pasty looking. They called the hospital and got a room ready for me. I went home and packed the usual bag of essentials for probably another week in the hospital and called Tony. He was on his way home from work and said that he would take me. I called my mom and dad and told them the wonderful news. Then, I called my boss and explained what was happening. He was good about it and said to keep him informed.

So, I get to my room and it turns out that I am sharing it with someone who has to have camera surveillance. I found out that she had some form of mental retardation and needed to be monitored for her safety. How could I find out such information when we have the Privacy Act???? Anyway, her family would bring in fast food for ALL three meals and she would eat it AND her meal tray from the dietary department!! Turns out, she also had diabetes, was overweight and had a kidney problem. Her family had no problem sharing this information with me. Imagine how I felt, smelling all of that wonderful food. It's not good for you, but it sure smelled good! I was jealous.

Anyway, one of the first things they do after you put on the fashionable gown, is to put in an IV line for fluids. It took three nurses to hit a vein. I was so dehydrated that my veins were flat. Once the line was in, they drew some blood to check my electrolytes and other blood chemistries. Initially, they hooked up a liter of Normal Saline. This would change once the results of my labs came back. Not even half way through the first bag, it was changed to include potassium. I was low in potassium, sodium, chloride and glucose.

Being a nurse, as well as an advocate for my health, I asked my doctor if I could see the labs for myself. My primary care physician has never had a problem with me looking at my test results. Sure enough, my white blood cells were elevated, my hemoglobin was low, albumin was low, platelets were elevated and my red blood cells were slightly low. That explains my beautiful skin color!

The next day, I noticed that my arm was starting to burn and form a red line from where the IV was traveling. I reported this to my nurse and asked her to turn down the rate of infusion because I was having a sensitivity to the potassium. This is very common. Potassium burns a lot of people if infused too quickly. My IV was going at 125ml/hr. The doctor responded pretty quick and said to lower it to 100ml/hr and see if that helped. I said that I would try to tolerate it as much as possible because I knew the importance of maintaining a normal level of potassium.

The same day, a new GI doc entered my life. I will not name him because I did not like him. I did not appreciate the way he spoke down to me. He immediately said that I needed a feeding tube and basically that is all he said. He was in and out so fast. He was picked to see me because if you remember, my GI doc is in Philly. The hospital just assigned him to me. Lucky me. Once he left, I asked for my primary physician to be called. I was told that he would be making rounds soon and to hang in there. Great answer.

When my primary came in later that day, we had a long chat about my current condition and how I am going to adopt a child and take care of him when I am so sick. We had a true and real conversation about the feeding tube. I told him that I would consider it and I will let him know in the morning. I really needed to sleep on it at this point. It was a lot to handle. First of all, Tony and I were getting closer to going to China for our little boy. Second, how was I going to handle such a trip feeling like this? How was I going to handle a trip with a feeding tube?

Well, when my family came in to see me, I told them what both doctors had said regarding the tube and they seemed concerned and agreed. My mother, especially, wanted me to get stronger. She told me that right now, this is what my body needs and I need to listen to my body and get healthy. Those were not her exact words, but you get the picture.

I had a long night that night. I could not fall asleep. I kept thinking about all of the variables that go along with the tube feeding. Remember that I had one previously and I did NOT ENJOY IT! But, my main reason to agree to it was that there was a three year old boy waiting for me in China. He needed a mother and father. He needed a mother.

The next morning, I asked my nurse to call my primary and request a surgical consult with the same doctor who removed my gallbladder, Dr. Peter Andrews. My doctor immediately agreed and the surgeon was called. That evening, Dr. Andrews came in to see me and assess the situation. We talked for a while about my current health, the pending adoption and my future health. He looked at my abdomen and we discussed where the tube was going to be placed and told me that he would schedule the surgery for the next day!

My family came in shortly after the surgeon and I told them about the surgical plan. I was feeling nervous having to go through this again. I also had to call my boss and tell him that I would be out of work for another week, depending upon my recovery. My boss was very good with the news and told me to take my time and recover appropriately. As always, I acted calm and collected in front of my family. I kept up the façade that everything was alright and that I was not scared. Truth be told, I was and still am afraid for my life and what my future holds---everyday. It is amazing how your priorities shift and your thought process changes once you are faced with your own mortality.

Surgery day. Again. The escorts came to my room to wheel me down to the operating room early in the morning. My IV line needed to be changed due to the rules and regulations regarding time frames of IV's. Once this was done, I was ready to "go under", again.

I remember nothing about this procedure except that I woke up. Good sign. Again, there was a huge bandage around my entire mid-section. Not a lot of pain. Just a little discomfort. I had the usual dry mouth and requested mouth swabs and water. I did this for a few hours until I was able to get rid of the dryness and actually drink something. Not new to surgery, I knew the importance of ambulating as soon as possible afterwards to prevent blood clots and to aerate my lungs. So, after a brief rest, I remember my mother helping me up and going for a walk around the nurse's station with me. She helped me to balance my IV pole as well as balance ME. I was still a little woozy from the anesthesia.

Getting back in bed was always the fun part. I did my signature move of getting into the bed on my knees and sliding to my back. Sounds goofy, but it worked the best for me. I managed to sleep pretty good that night. Probably because the anxiety of the surgery was over. Morning came and my doctor and the surgeon came in to see me. They told me the usual routine of being able to eat ANYTHING and the ability to use the bathroom will buy me my discharge ticket. I ate most of the clear liquid tray and was able to use the bathroom without any problems except for the amount of time it took me to get there!

While I was waiting for the discharge instructions to be written, I called my husband and told him that I was getting ready to come home. As I waited for him, I got myself washed up and dressed and kept on ambulating in the halls.

Once settled at home, the delivery came to my house with the formula and all of the other goodies like the first time. I was going to do my feedings via gravity and not by pump this time. I was not on the schedule for 12 hour feeds. I was told to give myself 1-2 cans three times a day, more if I was vomiting. I refused the home health nurse this time because I felt confident enough to handle it, again.

Things were going pretty good with the feeding tube and I was using it three times a day and flushing it before and after usage. I was eating a little bit better. Cereal, eggs, toast and yogurt.

After a few more days of rest, I was ready to return to work. With my pole and feeding supplies in hand, I walked into my office. I received a lot of mixed greetings. People just didn't know how to approach me. I think it was quite an adjustment for them as well as for me. Every morning, there would be a department head meeting and it so happens that it was at the time when my feeding was due. I would hook myself up and drag my pole to the conference room. In the beginning, everyone would stare out of curiosity and wonderment. I took a few moments to explain to everyone that it was ok and that I am fine and I just want to keep working. A few of the upper management were concerned that I could not do my job while being connected to a feeding tube. They expressed this to me and I have to say that I was extremely disappointed. These are members of the healthcare community and they were acting as if there was not a compassionate bone in their bodies.

I had the opportunity to prove them all wrong. One day, I was walking in the hall with my feeding running when a client collapsed in front of me. As a nurse, my first response is always patient safety. I clamped off my tube feeding, called out for help and began CPR. I don't remember if it hurt, I only remember that my responsibility was to that client who was unresponsive. A few of my co-workers appeared and we all took turns continuing CPR until the 911 crew arrived. We managed to get him stable enough for transport to the hospital. Unfortunately, he expired shortly after getting to the ER. We were told it was due to a massive heart attack.

Upon seeing me in action, my boss approached me and apologized for ever having doubted me and my nursing abilities. I briefly said "Thank You" and walked away and continued my tube feeding.

The feedings were going pretty good, but I woke up one day and had unrelenting pain every time I touched the tube. I went to work not thinking much of it until I saw some green drainage and little bit of blood. I knew this was a sign to call the surgeon. Infection. I left work immediately and went to the surgeon's office. He injected my abdomen with Lidocaine to numb the area and removed the tube. All I remember seeing was an extremely long tube covered with green gunk and blood. The surgeon then covered the area with a bandage and explained to me the importance of drinking the tube feeding formula to maintain my nutritional status. If you have any experience with tube feed formulas, you know they STINK!

Now my diet consists of cereal, eggs, toast, yogurt and yummy tube feeding formula! I tried to add some chocolate powder to it to give it some taste. That did not turn out so good. I also tried to freeze some and make shakes and smoothies. YUCK! So in the end, I bit the bullet and just drank it straight. I tried to block it out of my mind because I knew my body really needed the nutrition. I have kept and still keep it at work so that I am fully prepared when my body needs it.

# Chapter Twenty: My miracle.

We finally receive notification that we were going to travel to China on November 17, 2007 to officially meet and adopt our SON! After three long years of waiting, our dream was finally coming true. With the feeding tube removed, I was drinking the formula to help maintain my electrolytes. My husband told me that we were taking some of the formula with us so that I don't get sick in China.

In the time we were preparing for our trip, I was so excited that I didn't really think about being sick. I was so ready to meet my son! We did pack almost two weeks worth of formula for our stay in China. We also packed a whole bunch of clothes and some toys that we bought for our son, Dylan.

The whole trip to China was absolutely amazing and that could take up a whole other book!! We flew out of JFK in New York to LA and from LA to China. The whole trip took 21 hours!!!! When we landed in China, we met our guide and away to the orphanage we went. It's funny, with such a time difference, we did not experience jet lag. Maybe it was due to the extreme excitement we were feeling!

When we got to the orphanage, we had to go into a conference area first and complete the paperwork, lots of it. Then, they took us to the room where Dylan and other children were playing. When we first saw him, I could not stop crying. I could not believe that this was the little boy from the photos the agency had sent. All of the children came running over to us, except for him. He stayed away and just watched and studied us. We had brought some toys with us for Dylan and the other children were so excited that we just left those toys with them. We saved a few extra things for Dylan on the side.

One of the workers there brought Dylan out to the conference area and we spent a few minutes getting to know him before we were taken away by our guide. They got us settled in our car and handed Dylan to Tony. Dylan was crying for a while and stopped when the worker handed him some snacks. The boy loves to eat!!!

Long story short, we stayed in China for almost two weeks to complete the adoption. I drank my formula like a good girl and wouldn't you know, Dylan loved it! Truth be told, I was not feeling my best. However, the sheer joy of my new title helped me to forget all about gastroparesis. At least, while we were in China.

Adoption final and we fly home. Both sets of grandparents were beyond excited to meet the newest member of our family! Dylan was the first and remains the only grandchild for my parents. Tony has a sister who has two children. I can not begin to tell you how much LIFE this child has injected into all of us. I, personally, feel honored to have met him and now I am honored to call him my son.

That is all I choose to say about the adoption because I really could go on and on and I would not want to inadvertently exploit my son. Please understand.

# Chapter Twenty-One:
## The last surgery

Motherhood is going great and I would not change a thing, except for my current health status. I am always doing research for the latest and greatest in treatment options. I was doing a search on the web for doctors in my area who treat gastroparesis when I came upon a site for Dr. Clark Gerhart. This popped up because he performs the gastric pacemaker surgery. The site included his e-mail and I thought I would take a chance and send him a brief history of my eight year battle with this illness. To my surprise, he got back to me rather quickly and asked me to call his office for an appointment and we could discuss my situation.

About two weeks later, I was in his office. At first, we discussed the gastric pacer for the THIRD time. We decided to try it one more time because the other two options he had for me were a "modified" gastric bypass and a gastrectomy. I, of course, wanted to try the lesser of the invasive procedures. Back to the drawing board with the insurance company. They rejected me. They told me it was not medically necessary. I then drafted a letter to my insurance company and described my daily life to them along with all of the treatments I had endured. They apparently did not care because I didn't receive a response.

Then, I called the doctor and asked for an appointment to discuss the other two options. At this point, I was leaning more towards the bypass procedure. My rationale that led me to that decision was the fact that with the pacer, I would need to get the battery replaced every 7-10 years. Can my body really handle surgery every 7-10 years as I age?

So, I did my homework on the bypass procedure and went in to this appointment with my questions in hand. Dr. Gerhart took his time and answered every question and calmed every fear that I had. I left his office feeling totally confident in his ability as a surgeon, his knowledge as a physician and his bedside manner as an empathetic human being.

Surgery was scheduled for October 3 and wouldn't you know, the insurance company had no problems approving this. Go figure! I am surprised because I am not obese and they did not question why I was going for this procedure. Oh well. I really couldn't think of that now. I was about to have a life changing surgery that could possibly "cure" my gastroparesis?? I started to wonder what it would be like to eat like a normal person again. What does an apple taste like? I have not had one in eight years and that is one of the first foods that I can't wait to taste! Well, I can't wait to taste it and swallow it and digest it! That is the most critical piece of all. Will it stay down and nourish my body? I know, one step at a time.

The procedure was technically a gastric bypass with a small bowel resection. The one thing that made my procedure different from the bariatric version was the size of the pouch to be created by the surgeon. He was going to create a larger pouch due to the fact that I did not need to lose weight. He was then going to literally bypass the lower 2/3 of my stomach and a portion of my small intestine and then reconnect the intestine to the "new" stomach and also reconnect the intestines at the lower end to form a "y". To find pictures of this procedure, just type in gastric bypass into any search engine. The procedure is so common now that I will not get into the details of it. I would rather speak on how it made me feel and how it has interfaced with the gastroparesis and my quality of life.

So, I went through the routine of pre-admission testing about one week prior to the surgery. I also went to the dentist and got my hair done the week before also. Why not go to the hospital all primped and preened!? It was actually just a coincidence.

The night before the surgery I did not sleep well. I was mostly concerned about my son adjusting to me not being there. If you remember, we adopted him on November 19 and this is not yet a full year for him. Tony and I decided that he should not come to see me in the hospital because of the NG tube, IV tube and various drains that I was going to have post-op. We did not want to scare him. He is currently obsessed with ambulances, fire trucks and police cars and we want him to keep his love for them and to continue his understanding that they help people.

Surgery day. I needed to be at the hospital around 10am. My husband stayed home with Dylan so that he could get him off to school. My mother and father drove me to the hospital and my brother met us there. I checked in to the short stay procedure unit and was assigned to my temporary bed. I changed into the beautiful gown and awaited the nurse for the IV and vital signs and the usual review of my health history.

With an IV in place and my family at my bedside, the surgeon appeared to answer any last minute questions. At this point, I was a little nervous. Not due to the procedure, due to the NG tube. It was and still is one of my greatest medical fears. I just don't like them. It seems unnatural! You remember my previous story about them?! After the surgeon left, the anesthesiologist came in to discuss the procedure and side effects of anesthetics. I had a patch on the back of one ear and I was told that they would hang Zofran for me in the O.R. I have the wonderful side effect of projectile vomiting upon waking up and with an NG tube, I did not want to vomit and create pressure and have it come out. Because if it comes out, it will go back in WHILE I AM AWAKE!

A few moments later, a nurse anesthetist came in to talk to me and then gave me some wonderful sleepy-time medicine. I think it only took a matter of seconds because I do not remember anything after the medicine was put in the IV.

Surgery was a success! Dr. Gerhart told my family that everything went very well and he was pleased with the result. I do not remember if I woke up in the recovery area due to the heavy dose of medications. I vaguely remember transferring to my bed in my room from the O.R. bed. I basically do not remember October 3. I really did not wake up until the next day. Even then, I was extremely groggy. My family was there at my bedside, so they say. I do not remember. I do remember one visit where I said that I was just going to close my eyes for a little while. I guess that turned into all night, because I did not wake up until the next day.

Friday was the surgery. Saturday, I slept off and on all day. I did notice that I had an NG tube and 2 drains in my abdomen along with 4 areas where steri-strips were. I was very lucky to have had the procedure through the laparascope. This makes for easier healing and moving around. Stubborn as I am, I was getting out of bed to use the bathroom almost every hour. I understand the importance of ambulation after surgery due to blood clots and I did not want any more problems! So, almost to the hour, I would ring for the nurse to help me with the NG, drains and my IV. Actually, I just needed the nurse to remove the NG from the wall suction and I would take the rest of it myself.

The wall suction was attached to the NG tube to make sure that my stomach remained empty so that healing could begin. At first, the contents were bright red blood. Over the three days it was in, it changed to dark brown, then green. I was not eating anything while the NG tube was in. I still had the continuous IV. Yummy.

On Sunday, I went to radiology for a barium study to check for leaks at the suture sites. They put barium mixed with water in a syringe and flushed my NG tube to verify that everything was ok. Once the radiologist saw the images on the screen, he assured me that all of the sutures were in tact and that there were no leaks!!! This was great news for me. It meant that the NG tube could come out! I just had to wait for the surgeon to come in and see the report.

Not long after I returned to my room from this test, the surgeon was in to see me. He told me that everything "looked good so far" and "let's get that tube out of your nose". He unwrapped the tape that held it in place and before I could take a breath, it was out! What a wonderful relief. I immediately had to blow my nose and it was bleeding a little bit. This was normal due to the irritation. It felt so good to have one less tube holding me down. Keep in mind that I still had the two drains in my abdomen.

The surgeon examined me and said that it was time to try clear liquids. Are we having fun yet? I get to have jello, tea and broth. This is also what I had to eat for two weeks after the surgery to allow the healing process to continue. While I waited for my lunch tray, I washed up and went for a walk around the nurses' station. I felt so much better walking without that NG tube.

My meals are staying down and I am actually feeling pretty good. Tired and hungry, but good. The next day, the surgeon comes in and examines me again and reports that the drains can come out. I didn't even know what was happening because he did it so fast. All I felt was pressure for about ½ second and they were both out! The only tube I had left in me was the IV. I was thrilled to be even more mobile without the worry of the drains getting caught on something. Then the surgeon told me that I could go home the next day!!! I continued to enjoy my clear liquids and rested for one more day.

The day of discharge felt so good to me. The only challenge was going to be maintaining the clear liquid diet while my family would be enjoying delicious and savory solid foods! Well, that's a little dramatic. If I waited eight years for this moment, I certainly could wait a couple more weeks. Along with the clear liquids, I was told to get a multivitamin, vitamin B-12, calcium, vitamin D and folic acid. This is going to help with the nutrient deficiencies that I will be dealing with since the manipulation of the small bowel.

When I got home, I just wanted to pick up my son and hug him for hours. However, I could only hug him sitting down because I was restricted to less than 25 pounds. My son was so curious about the whole situation. He wanted to see my belly and I showed it to him. He still calls it my "boo-boo belly". He was not afraid to see the steri-strips or the swelling. He even got to the point of having broth with me. I think he missed me not eating with him.

So, two weeks go by and it is time for my first follow-up visit with the surgeon. I had lost some weight. This was to be expected due to the procedure and the fact that I had not eaten a solid, calorie laden meal in over two weeks. The surgeon was extremely pleased by how well I was doing. He told me that we will keep an eye on the weight loss. He also said that I could advance my diet to soft, finely chopped and pureed foods. This meant that I could now have scrambled eggs with my broth! He also told me to be patient because it could take up to three months for my insides to heal and be ready for "real" food. I am still not able to eat fiber, yet. The surgeon told me that maybe for Christmas I could have my apple!

I reported to him that I have NOT vomited since the surgery and that I considered the procedure to be 100% successful! He was very satisfied with that outcome. He then explained to me the feelings that I would get as I introduced food back into my system. I was told to eat very small portions. Approximately one cup of food at a time. I was to do this about five to six times a day. If I felt any discomfort, I was to stop eating and drink clear liquids, preferably a cup of hot tea to help break down the food that may or may not be stuck. He said that sometimes if the food is not broken down enough it could get stuck. So far, I have had that feeling a few times. It had gone away once I drank the hot tea.

I received permission from him to go back to work. Let me re-phrase that. I told him that I was ready to go back to work and please give me a note allowing me to do just that. My colleagues were surprised to see me so soon after the procedure. They knew what I was getting done and could not believe it when they saw me. They were and remain very supportive of my current diet restrictions and are looking forward to me eating "normally".

It has now been six weeks after the surgery and I feel good. I am not vomiting. I am not in pain. I am not nauseous. I am not taking ANY stomach meds, only my vitamins. Of course, I have early satiety because I need to adjust the quantity of food that I eat. I have not gained any weight back, yet. I know that will come in time.

My six week follow up with the surgeon was another success. He is so pleased with the results I am experiencing. I am also completely satisfied with the way I am feeling at this point. Thank you a thousand times over, Dr. Gerhart!! I am now upgraded to a regular diet. However, I need to go slow at first with the fruits and veggies. For starters, I can eat cooked veggies, not raw. I can eat an apple, without the skin. As for lettuce, I will have to chop that up finely if I would like a salad. I think I will wait a couple more months before I try that.

My labs are being followed carefully and so far, I am doing well. No major abnormalities. I am also allowed to exercise again.

Of course, I have to take it easy due to the fact that I do not want to lose any more weight. I will start off with maybe three days a week for about half an hour and see how it goes. I really want to focus on building up my strength.

I can now sit back, continue my recovery and enjoy the holidays with my family and friends. I will see the surgeon again in three months for a check-up. This may be the first Christmas in years that I might be able to enjoy the TASTE of food without the worry of gastroparesis rearing its ugly head! Notice that I said the TASTE of food and not eating the food. When you lose the ability to eat and enjoy the textures, flavors and tastes of things, it all gets put into perspective. I do not take eating and digestion for granted. I am now in a place where I appreciate what food can do for my body. I have been watching the Food Network like crazy coming up with new ideas for dishes I was never able to tolerate.

# Chapter Twenty-Two:
# The future

I wish I knew where the trend in gastroparesis care was going. I, personally, have tried all of the latest treatments. The gastric bypass is really something new in the treatment of gastroparesis. When I think about the illness and my current age of 38, the future sometimes frightens me. When I have a good day, I run with it. Bad days, I wish would hurry and go away. I try to think positive, but it does get hard when you try all of the latest therapies and they fail for you. I was told by a handful of doctors to have a total gastrectomy in response to all of the other treatment failures. This I will not allow unless it is truly considered a matter of "life or death". Once your stomach is removed, it can't magically come back or be replaced. I guess that is another reason why I chose bypass.

I will continue to see my specialist in Philadelphia, Dr. Robert Fisher. I will look into every clinical trial that comes down the pike and see if I would benefit by enrolling. I will do my best to maintain a positive attitude for me and my family. I want to be a role model for my son and others who are suffering with this disease. I want to raise awareness that gastroparesis is alive and well in this country and currently has no cure. Although, the gastric bypass has had many positive outcomes from those who have had it done, myself included. I am not sure at this point if I would say the word cure, but perhaps remission?

I will say that I am grateful for my husband, Tony. He has endured a lot with me. Especially for a guy who really hates medicine. I give him a lot of credit for seeing me through the difficult times.

I am grateful to have my mother and father by my side. My father is the kind of guy that wants to fix things if they are broken and he did not know how to fix me. I know that this frustrated him, but what was most important to me is that he never gave up on me and was always there when I needed his support.

My mother deserves special mention because she has gone on almost every appointment and to every procedure. Tony, due to his work schedule, could not always get the time off. My mother was, and still is, my driver when I get sedated for EGD's. She is my friend when I need to complain about this disease. But most of all, she is and always will be my mom! She has always dropped everything to care for me and made sure that I had what I needed. I could never thank her enough.

Finally, for those of you suffering with gastroparesis, stay strong, stay focused and never stop looking for that silver lining. It is out there and it took me eight years of trial and error procedures to find it. I have never let the illness get in the way of achieving my goals. It may have blocked them, but only temporarily. Today, I emerge a stronger and more perceptive person. Dare I say, I owe it all to gastroparesis?

14137214R00079

Made in the USA
Lexington, KY
11 March 2012